LOSE BACK FAT

FAT

Easy exercise workout to reduce back fat

Doris A. Freema

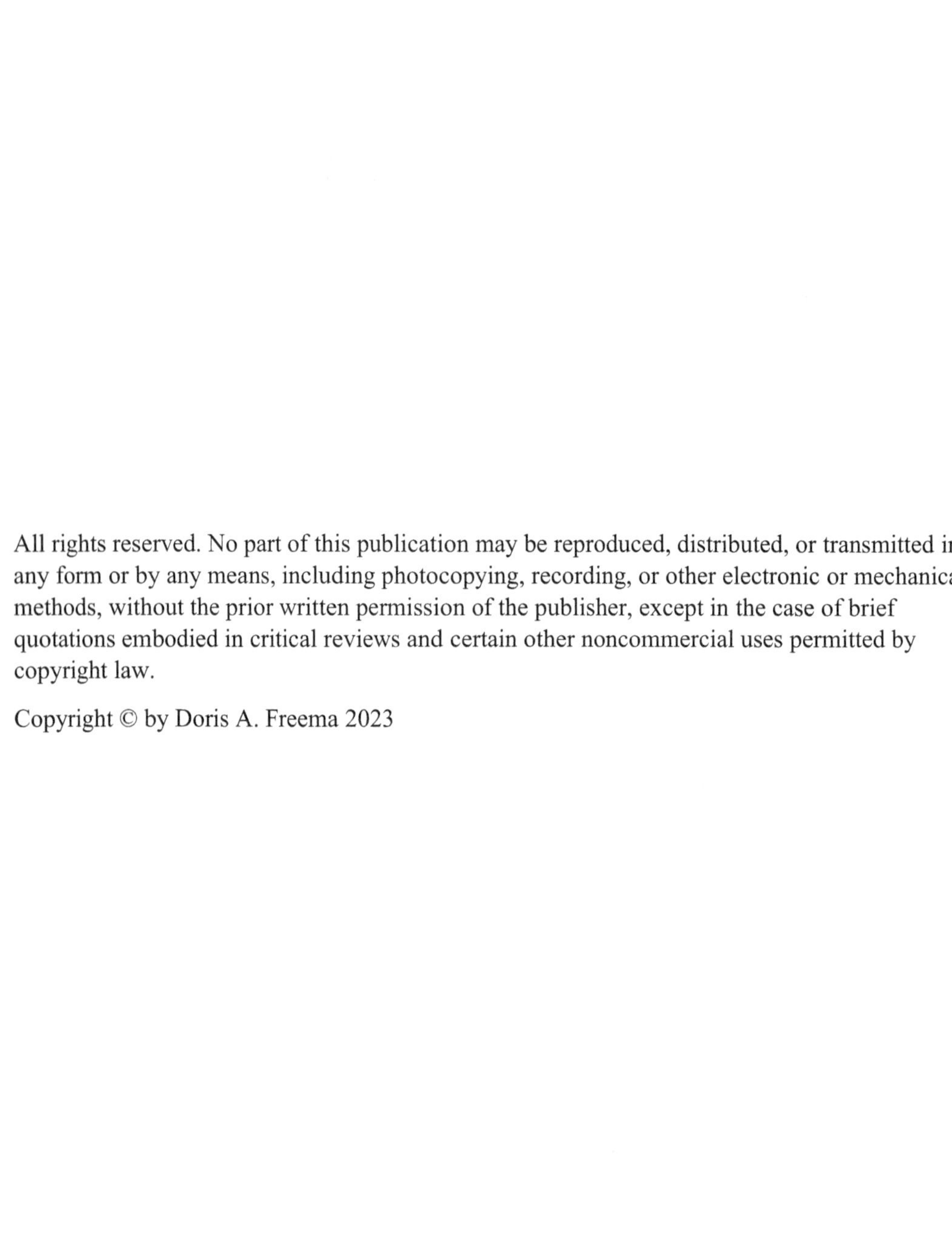

Table of content

INTRODUCTION

CHAPTER ONE

Importance of reducing back fat for overall health

CHAPTER TWO

Easy exercise workout for reducing back fat

CHAPTER THREE

Neck rotations and shoulder rolls to loosen up the upper

Body

CHAPTER FOUR

Gentle back stretches to prepare the muscles for the workout

CHAPTER FIVE

Light cardiovascular exercise like jogging in place or jumping jacks to increase heart rate

CHAPTER SIX

Upper back exercises: rows, reverse fly, and lat pulldowns

CHAPTER SEVEN

Lower back exercises: supermans bridges and bird dogs

CHAPTER EIGHT

Core exercises: planks, side planks, and Russian twists to strengthen the abdominal muscles and support the back

CHAPTER NINE

Cardiovascular exercises for overall fat burning/ high intensity interval training (HIIT) workouts to maximize calorie burn

CHAPTER TEN

Incorporating aerobic activities into daily routines, such as brisk walking or stair climbing

CHAPTER ELEVEN

Cool down and stretching exercises

INTRODUCTION

Back fat, also known as dorsal fat, refers to the accumulation of excess adipose tissue or fat in the area of the back. This can manifest as visible bulges, folds, or thicknesses in the upper and lower back regions. Back fat can be a source of concern for some individuals due to aesthetic reasons or potential health implications. It often becomes more noticeable when wearing certain types of clothing or swimwear, and it may affect an individual's self-confidence.

Causes of Back Fat:

The development of back fat is primarily influenced by factors related to an individual's lifestyle, genetics, and overall health. Some common causes and contributing factors include:

Dietary Habits: A diet high in calories, unhealthy fats, and sugar can lead to weight gain and the accumulation of fat throughout the body, including the back. Consuming more calories than the body requires can result in the storage of excess energy as fat.

Lack of Physical Activity: Sedentary lifestyles and insufficient physical activity can lead to weight gain and the accumulation of fat in various areas of the body, including the back. Regular exercise helps burn calories and maintain healthy body composition.

Genetics: Genetic factors play a role in determining an individual's body shape, fat distribution, and propensity to gain weight in certain areas. Some people may be genetically predisposed to storing fat in the back region.

Changes in hormones: this takes place during puberty, pregnancy, and menopause, and can affect fat distribution. Hormonal imbalances can lead to increased fat storage in certain areas, including the back.

As we age individually, our metabolism slows down, and muscle mass decreases. This can result in a gradual increase in body fat, including back fat.

Stress: Chronic stress can lead to the overproduction of cortisol, a hormone that can promote fat storage, particularly in the abdominal and back areas.

Poor Posture: Maintaining poor posture can lead to muscle imbalances and the appearance of back fat. Slouching and hunching can cause the skin and underlying tissues to fold and bunch up, creating the appearance of excess fat.

Lack of Muscle Tone: Weak back muscles can contribute to the accumulation of fat in the back area. Developing and maintaining muscle tone through strength training can help improve the overall appearance of the back.

It's important to note that spot reduction, which involves targeting specific areas of the body for fat loss through exercise, is generally not a practical approach. Instead, adopting a balanced and healthy lifestyle that includes a well-rounded diet, regular physical activity, and stress management can contribute to overall fat loss and improve body composition, including reducing back fat over time.

CHAPTER ONE

Importance of reducing back fat for overall health

Reducing back fat is not just about improving physical appearance; it also holds important implications for overall health. Excess fat accumulation, particularly in the back region, can have various negative effects on health and well-being. Here are some reasons why reducing back fat is important for overall health:

Cardiovascular Health: Excess fat, especially in the upper back and around the waist, is associated with an increased risk of cardiovascular diseases such as heart disease and hypertension. This type of fat, known as visceral fat, releases inflammatory substances that can contribute to the development of arterial plaque and increase the risk of heart-related issues.

Metabolic Health: Accumulation of fat in the back and other areas can lead to insulin resistance and metabolic syndrome, both of which are risk factors for type 2 diabetes. Improving body composition through fat reduction can help enhance insulin sensitivity and metabolic health.

Joint and Musculoskeletal Health: Carrying excess weight in the back can strain the spine, leading to poor posture and discomfort. This can result in musculoskeletal issues, back pain, and increased stress on the joints. Reducing back fat can alleviate some of these issues and promote better spine alignment.

Respiratory Function: Excessive fat around the chest and upper back can affect lung capacity and respiratory function. This can lead to reduced oxygen intake, decreased lung efficiency, and potentially hindered physical performance.

Hormonal Balance: Fat tissue can produce hormones and other bioactive molecules that influence hormonal balance. Reducing excess fat can help promote hormonal equilibrium, which is important for various bodily functions, including reproductive health and stress regulation.

Self-Esteem and Mental Health: While physical health is crucial, mental and emotional well-being are equally important. Experiencing dissatisfaction with one's appearance due to back fat can impact self-esteem and body image. Working on fat reduction and achieving fitness goals can boost self-confidence and contribute to better mental health.

Long-Term Weight Management: Addressing back fat is part of a comprehensive approach to weight management. By adopting healthier lifestyle habits, such as balanced nutrition and regular exercise, individuals can better maintain a healthy weight in the long run.

Inflammation and Chronic Diseases: Excess fat in the body can contribute to chronic low-level inflammation, which is linked to various chronic diseases, including cancer. By reducing back fat and overall body fat, individuals can help lower their risk of developing these diseases.

CHAPTER TWO

Easy exercise workout for reducing back fat

Engaging in regular exercise is essential for reducing back fat and improving overall health. Cardiovascular exercise, strength training, and flexibility work can help target this area effectively. Here's a simple workout routine that you can follow to help reduce back fat:

Warm-Up:

To increase blood circulation in the body, begin with a 5-10 min warm-up. With light exercises.

Cardiovascular Exercise (20-30 minutes):

To promote fat loss engaging in cardiovascular exercises burns more calories. Choose activities you enjoy, such as brisk walking, jogging, cycling, swimming, or dancing. Aim for 20-30 minutes of continuous activity at a moderate intensity.

Strength Training (3 times per week):

Strength training helps build muscle mass, increase metabolism, and improve overall body composition. Focus on exercises that target the back muscles, as well as other major muscle groups. Here's a simple strength training routine:

Push-Ups: Perform 3 sets of 10-15 repetitions. Push-ups engage the chest, shoulders, and upper back muscles.

Bent-Over Rows: Use dumbbells or resistance bands. Perform 3 sets of 12-15 repetitions. This singles out the middle and upper back muscles.

Lat Pulldowns: If you have access to a gym or a resistance band, lat pulldowns are excellent for targeting the upper back. Perform 3 sets of 10-12 repetitions.

Superman: Lie face down on the floor. Raise your arms and legs off the ground simultaneously, engaging your lower back muscles. Hold for a few seconds and release. Do 3 sets of 12-15 repetitions.

Flexibility and Cool Down:

After your strength training, spend a few minutes stretching the back muscles and other major muscle groups. Gentle stretches help improve flexibility and prevent muscle tightness.

Kick off with weights that dare you but support proper form. Gently multiply the weight as you progress.

Drink water before and after a workout to stay hydrated.

Balanced Diet: Focus on a balanced diet that includes lean proteins, whole grains, healthy fats, and various fruits and vegetables.

Consistency: Consistency is vital to seeing results. Make working out a part of your life.

Rest: Rest between workout sessions allows recovery before the next workout. This is for muscle repairs and growth.

Always listen to yourself during exercise. if you feel uncomfortable during an exercise, stop immediately.

Gradual Progression: As you become more comfortable, consider increasing the intensity, duration, or frequency of your workouts to continue challenging your body.

Remember that spot reduction is not guaranteed, but a comprehensive exercise routine combined with a healthy lifestyle can help you achieve your fitness and fat loss goals, including reducing back fat over time.

CHAPTER THREE

Neck rotations and shoulder rolls to loosen up the upper Body

Warming up is crucial before engaging in any exercise routine, as it helps prevent injuries and prepares your body for more intense physical activity.

Neck Rotations:

Neck rotations help release tension and improve flexibility in the neck and upper back area.

Sit up straight and ease your shoulders.

Gently tilt your head to the right, bringing your right ear towards your right shoulder.

Hold the stretch for a few seconds, feeling a gentle stretch along the left side of your neck.

Slowly return to the center and repeat the tilt to the left side.

Continue alternating sides for 8-10 rotations on each side.

Shoulder Rolls:

Shoulder rolls help improve shoulder mobility and release tension in the upper back and shoulders.

Stand up straight with your arms relaxed by your sides.

Slowly roll your shoulders in a circular motion, moving them forward.

Complete 8-10 forward rolls and then reverse the motion.

Roll your shoulders in a circular motion moving them backward for 8-10 repetitions.

Remember to perform these warm-up exercises in a controlled and gentle manner. The goal is to gradually increase blood flow to the muscles and joints without causing any strain. After completing these exercises, you should feel more limber and ready for your main workout.

As always, listen to your body and adjust the intensity of the warm-up based on your comfort level. If you have any pre-existing medical conditions or concerns, it's a good idea to consult with a healthcare professional before starting a new exercise routine.

CHAPTER FOUR

Gentle back stretches to prepare the muscles for the workout

Gentle back stretches can help prepare your muscles for a workout by increasing blood flow, improving flexibility, and reducing the risk of injury.

Cat-Cow Stretch:

In a tabletop position. Start on your hands and knees

Inhale, arch your back and lift your head and tailbone (cow pose).

Exhale, round your back, tuck your chin to your chest and engage your core (cat pose).

The flow between cat and cow poses, moving with your breath, for 5-8 cycles.

Child's Pose:

Begin in a kneeling position with your big toes touching and knees apart.

Sit back onto your heels and extend your arms forward on the floor.

Rest your forehead on the ground and feel a gentle stretch in your lower back.

Hold for 20-30 seconds while taking deep breaths.

Seated Forward Fold:

Sit on the floor with your legs extended in front of you.

Hinge at your hips and reach your hands toward your feet.

Keep your spine straight as you fold forward, feeling a stretch in your hamstrings and lower back.

Hold for 20-30 seconds and breathe deeply.

Spinal Twist:

Sit on the floor with your legs extended in front of you.

Bend your right knee and place your right foot outside your left thigh.

Gently twist to the right, placing your left elbow on the outside of your right knee and your right hand behind you.

Inhale to lengthen your spine, and exhale to deepen the twist.

Hold for 20-30 seconds, then switch sides.

Standing Forward Fold:

Stand with your feet hip-width apart.

Hinge at your hips and fold forward, letting your upper body hang down.

Bend your knees slightly if needed to keep your spine straight.

Feel the stretch in your entire back, from your neck to your lower back.

Hold for 20-30 seconds and breathe deeply.

Thread the Needle Stretch:

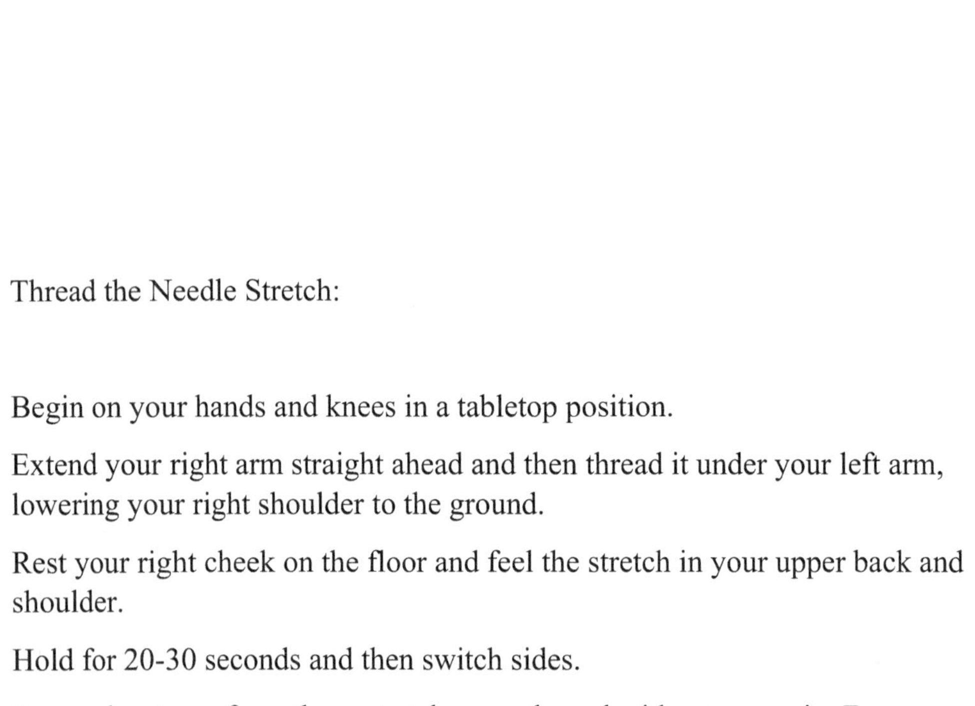

Begin on your hands and knees in a tabletop position.

Extend your right arm straight ahead and then thread it under your left arm, lowering your right shoulder to the ground.

Rest your right cheek on the floor and feel the stretch in your upper back and shoulder.

Hold for 20-30 seconds and then switch sides.

Remember to perform these stretches gently and without any pain. Focus on breathing deeply and relaxing into each stretch. These stretches will help prepare your back muscles for your workout and improve your overall flexibility.

CHAPTER FIVE

Light cardiovascular exercise like jogging in place or jumping jacks to increase heart rate

Incorporating light cardiovascular exercises into your warm-up routine is an excellent way to elevate your heart rate and prepare your body for more intense physical activity.

Jogging in Place:

Be with your feet hip-width apart and arms by your sides.

Lift your knees alternatively, as if you're jogging, while keeping your upper body relaxed.

Engage your core and swing your arms gently as you jog in place.

Aim to maintain a steady pace and breathe rhythmically.

Continue jogging in place for 2-3 minutes.

Jumping Jacks:

Begin with your feet jointly and arms by your sides.

At the same time, jump your feet apart and lift up your arms high up

Jump again to bring your feet back together while lowering your arms.

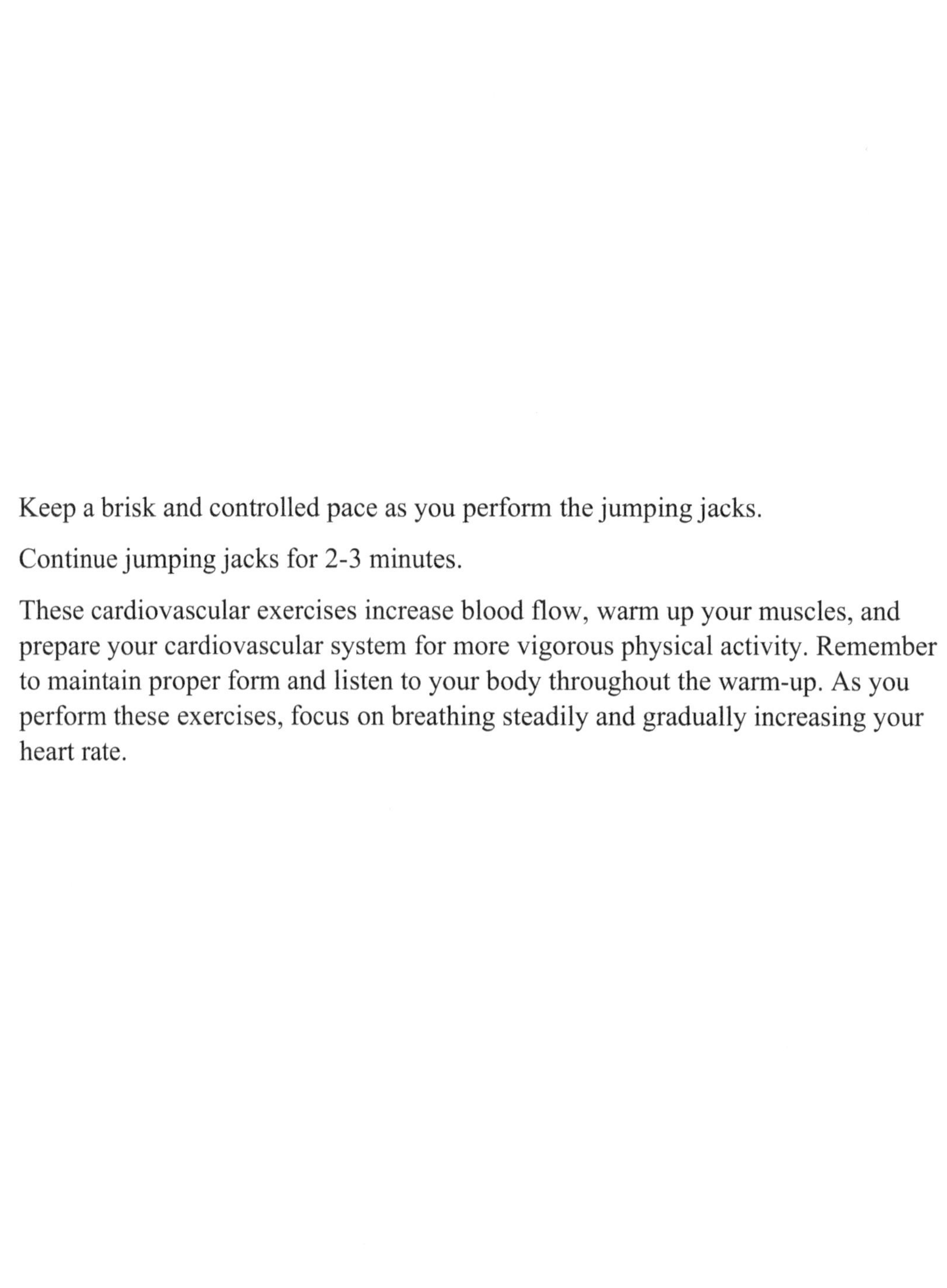

Keep a brisk and controlled pace as you perform the jumping jacks.

Continue jumping jacks for 2-3 minutes.

These cardiovascular exercises increase blood flow, warm up your muscles, and prepare your cardiovascular system for more vigorous physical activity. Remember to maintain proper form and listen to your body throughout the warm-up. As you perform these exercises, focus on breathing steadily and gradually increasing your heart rate.

CHAPTER SIX

Upper back exercises: rows, reverse fly, and lat pulldowns

Targeted exercises for the upper back can help strengthen the muscles in that area and contribute to back fat reduction over time. Here are three effective exercises you mentioned: rows, reverse flies, and lat pulldowns. These exercises focus on different aspects of the upper back and can be incorporated into your workout routine for better muscle definition and overall back strength:

Rows:

Equipment: Dumbbells, barbells, or resistance bands.

Technique:

Kickstart with your feet shoulder-width apart, knees a little bent.

Hold a dumbbell in each hand or grip the barbell with an overhand grip.

Depends on your hips, keeping your back aligned and chest up.

Bend your elbows and pull the weight(s) toward your lower ribs, squeezing your shoulder blades together.

Lower the weight(s) back down in a controlled manner.

Perform 3 sets of 10-12 repetitions.

Reverse Flies:

Equipment: Dumbbells.

Technique:

Hold a dumbbell in each hand and stand with your feet hip-width apart.

Depends on your hips, maintaining a slight bend in your knees.

Let the dumbbells hang in front of you, palms facing each other.

Keeping a slight bend in your elbows, lift your arms out to the sides until they're parallel to the ground.

Squeeze your shoulder blades together and pause briefly before lowering the weights.

Perform 3 sets of 12-15 repetitions.

Lat Pulldowns:

Equipment: Lat pulldown machine or resistance bands.

Technique:

Sit at the lat pulldown machine or attach resistance bands overhead.

Grip the bar or bands with a wide grip, hands facing forward.

Engage your core and pull the bar/bands down toward your chest while arching your back slightly.

Squeeze your shoulder blades together and pause at the bottom of the movement.

Slowly release the bar/bands back up to the starting position.

Perform 3 sets of 10-12 repetitions.

Incorporate these exercises into your strength training routine, focusing on proper form and gradually increasing the weight or resistance as you become more comfortable. Remember that spot reduction isn't guaranteed, so combining these exercises with a balanced diet, cardiovascular exercises, and a comprehensive fitness regimen will help you achieve your back fat reduction goals more effectively.

CHAPTER SEVEN

Lower back exercises: supermans bridges and bird dogs

These exercises can be beneficial for improving core stability and lower back strength. However, I'd like to provide a brief overview of how to perform these exercises correctly:

Superman Bridges:

Superman bridges target the lower back, glutes, and hamstrings.

How to do it:

a. Lie face down on an exercise mat or comfortable surface.

b. Extend your arms straight in front of you and keep your legs straight.

c. Simultaneously lift your arms, chest, and legs off the ground while contracting your lower back muscles.

d. Hold this position for a few seconds while keeping your core engaged.

e. Slowly lower your arms, chest, and legs back down to the ground.

Bird Dogs:

Bird Dogs are a great exercise for core stability and balance, which can indirectly help strengthen the lower back.

How to do it:

a. Kickstart with your hands and knees in a tabletop position.

b. Extend your right arm straight out in front of you while simultaneously extending your left leg straight back.

c. Keep your hips level and your core engaged to maintain stability.

d. Hold this position for a few seconds, focusing on keeping your body aligned.

e. Return your arm and leg to the starting position.

f. Repeat the movement on the opposite side, extending your left arm and right leg.

Remember to perform these exercises with proper form to avoid strain or injury. It's a good idea to consult a fitness professional or healthcare provider before starting a new exercise routine, especially if you have any pre-existing conditions or concerns about your lower back.

Additionally, these exercises can be incorporated into a broader workout routine that includes a variety of movements to target different muscle groups for overall strength and fitness.

CHAPTER EIGHT

Core exercises: planks, side planks, and Russian twists to strengthen the abdominal muscles and support the back

Planks: Planks are a fundamental core exercise that engages multiple muscle groups, including the abdominals, lower back, and shoulders. To perform a plank:

Kick-off in a push-up position with your hands straight under your shoulders.

Keep your body in a straight line from head to heels, engaging your core muscles to prevent your hips from sagging.

Hold this position for a specific duration, gradually increasing the time as your strength improves.

Side Planks: Side planks target the oblique muscles on the sides of your abdomen. They also engage the stabilizing muscles of your core and shoulders. This is how to do a side plank:

Lie on your side with your legs straight and feet stacked on top of each other.

Prop yourself up on your elbow, making sure it's directly under your shoulder.

Lift your hips off the ground, forming a straight line from your head to your feet.

Hold this position for a specific duration, then switch to the other side.

Russian Twists: Russian twists are a dynamic core exercise that involves twisting movements to engage the oblique and improve rotational strength. Here's how to perform them:

Sit on the floor with your knees bent and your feet flat.

Lean back slightly while maintaining a straight back.

Lift your feet off the ground, balancing on your sit bones.

Holding a weight or medicine ball, twist your torso to one side, bringing the weight toward the floor beside your hip.

Return to the center and then twist to the other side. That's one repetition.

Incorporating these exercises into your routine can help you develop a strong and stable core, which is crucial for maintaining proper posture, supporting your spine, and preventing back pain.

Remember to start with appropriate difficulty levels and gradually increase intensity and duration as your core strength improves. Always prioritize proper form to avoid injury. If you have any pre-existing medical conditions or concerns, it's a good idea to consult with a fitness professional or healthcare provider before starting a new exercise regimen.

CHAPTER NINE

Cardiovascular exercises for overall fat burning/ high intensity interval training (HIIT) workouts to maximize calorie burn

Cardiovascular exercises are great for overall fat burning, and high-intensity interval training (HIIT) is an effective method to maximize calorie burn and improve cardiovascular fitness. Here are some examples of both types of exercises:

Cardiovascular Exercises:

Running or Jogging: Running or jogging is a classic cardiovascular exercise that can be done outdoors or on a treadmill. It's effective for burning calories and improving endurance.

Cycling: Whether you're cycling on a stationary bike or on the road, cycling is a low-impact exercise that can be adapted to different fitness levels.

Swimming: Swimming is a full-body workout that engages various muscle groups while providing an excellent cardiovascular workout.

Jump Rope: Jumping rope is a simple yet effective way to get your heart rate up and burn calories. It can be done anywhere and anytime.

Rowing: Rowing machines provide a full-body workout that engages both upper and lower body muscles while giving you a solid cardiovascular challenge.

High-Intensity Interval Training (HIIT) Workouts:

HIIT involves alternating between periods of high-intensity exercise and periods of rest or low-intensity recovery. This approach can significantly boost calorie burn and improve cardiovascular fitness in a shorter amount of time.

Tabata Training: Tabata involves performing an exercise at maximum intensity for 20 seconds, followed by 10 seconds of rest. This cycle is repeated for a total of 4 minutes.

Sprint Intervals: On a track or a treadmill, alternate between sprinting at maximum effort for a certain distance or time, and then walking or jogging to recover.

Bodyweight HIIT: Create a circuit of bodyweight exercises (e.g., burpees, jumping jacks, mountain climbers, squat jumps) and perform each exercise for 30 seconds with 10-15 seconds of rest in between.

Circuit Training: Combine cardiovascular exercises with strength training exercises in a circuit format. For example, alternate between jump squats and push-ups for a set time before moving to the next exercise.

HIIT Classes: Many fitness classes and online workouts are dedicated to HIIT training. These classes often incorporate a variety of exercises and formats to keep the workout engaging.

Remember to warm up before starting any high-intensity workout, and cool down and stretch afterward. The intensity of your workouts should be tailored to your fitness level, and it's always a good idea to consult with a fitness professional or healthcare provider before starting a new exercise program.

CHAPTER TEN

Incorporating aerobic activities into daily routines, such as brisk walking or stair climbing

Incorporating aerobic activities like brisk walking and stair climbing into your daily routine is a fantastic way to improve your cardiovascular fitness and overall health.

Walking:

Walk Whenever Possible: Whenever you have the opportunity, choose walking over other modes of transportation, such as driving or taking the elevator.

Lunchtime Walks: Take a brisk walk during your lunch break. This can help you get some fresh air, clear your mind, and boost your energy for the afternoon.

Walking Meetings: If possible, schedule walking meetings with colleagues. This is a great way to combine work and physical activity.

Use a Pedometer or Fitness Tracker: Tracking your daily steps can motivate you to move more. Aim for a certain step goal and gradually increase it over time.

Stair Climbing:

Choose Stairs Over Elevators: Whenever you have the option, choose stairs instead of elevators or escalators. Climbing stairs is an excellent lower-body workout.

Stair Intervals: If you have access to a staircase, consider doing stair intervals. Climb the stairs at a brisk pace for a set number of flights, then recover on the way down.

Incorporate at Home: If you have stairs at home, use them as a workout tool. You can do step-ups, stair lunges, or simply walk up and down for a few minutes.

Tips for Success:

Start Slowly: If you're new to regular aerobic activity, start with manageable goals and gradually increase the duration and intensity of your walks and climbs.

Set a Schedule: Plan specific times for your aerobic activities and treat them like appointments. This helps ensure consistency.

Stay Hydrated: Carry a water bottle with you to stay hydrated during your walks and climbs, especially in hot weather.

Wear Comfortable Shoes: Proper footwear is essential for comfort and preventing injuries during walking and stair climbing.

Listen to Music or Podcasts: Create an enjoyable playlist or listen to podcasts during your walks to make the time more engaging.

Mix It Up: While brisk walking and stair climbing are great, it's also beneficial to incorporate a variety of aerobic activities to keep things interesting. This could include activities like cycling, swimming, dancing, or playing a sport you enjoy.

Progress Gradually: As your fitness improves, you can gradually increase the duration and intensity of your walks and climbs. This could involve adding more stairs, increasing your pace, or extending the distance you walk.

Remember that consistency is key. Even shorter bouts of aerobic activity throughout the day can add up and provide significant health benefits. Always consult with a healthcare professional before making significant changes to your exercise routine, especially if you have any underlying health conditions.

CHAPTER ELEVEN

Cool down and stretching exercises

Cooling down and stretching after your workouts is important for promoting flexibility, preventing muscle soreness, and aiding in your overall recovery.

Cool Down:

Walking or Slow Jogging: After an intense workout, gradually decrease your pace to a light walk or slow jog for a few minutes. This helps your heart rate return to its normal resting state.

Deep Breathing: Practice deep and controlled breathing to help relax your body and reduce stress.

Static Stretching: Gently stretch the muscles you worked during your workout. Hold each stretch for 15-30 seconds without bouncing. Some effective stretches include hamstring stretches, quad stretches, and calf stretches.

Stretching Exercises:

Hamstring Stretch: Sit on the ground with one leg extended and the other bent so your foot rests against the inner thigh of the extended leg. Reach forward toward your toes, keeping your back straight.

Quad Stretch: Stand on one leg and bend the other leg at the knee, bringing your foot toward your glutes. Hold your ankle and gently pull your foot closer to your glutes while keeping your knees together.

Calf Stretch: Find a wall or stable surface to lean against. Place one foot forward and one foot back, keeping your back leg straight and your heel on the ground. Lean forward to feel a stretch in your calf.

Hip Flexor Stretch: Take a lunge position with one foot forward and the other foot extended back. Gently push your hips forward while keeping your back straight to feel a stretch in the front of your hip.

Child's Pose: Start on your hands and knees, then sit back on your heels while extending your arms forward. This stretch targets your lower back and hips.

Triceps Stretch: Raise one arm overhead and bend your elbow so your hand reaches toward the opposite shoulder blade. Gently push down on the bent elbow with your opposite hand to feel a stretch in your triceps.

Shoulder Stretch: Extend one arm across your body at chest height. Use your opposite hand to gently pull your arm closer to your chest.

Seated Forward Fold: Sit with your legs extended in front of you. Hinge at your hips and reach forward, aiming to touch your toes or shins while keeping your back straight.

Remember that stretching should not be painful. You should feel a gentle stretch, but not to the point of discomfort or pain. Perform your stretches in a calm and controlled manner, focusing on your breathing and relaxing into each stretch. Regular stretching can improve flexibility and range of motion, so aim to incorporate it into your routine a few times per week.